Under the Weeping Willow

About Death and Dying

Gerlinde Debie-Millette

Printed in the United States of America by Lightning Source, Inc.

ISBN 978-01-937862-77-0
Library of Congress Control Number 2014939714

The author of this book does not dispense medical advice or prescribe the use of any technique as a form of treatment for physical, emotional or medical problems without the advice of a physician, either directly or indirectly. The intent of the author is only to offer information of a general nature to help the reader in their quest for emotional and spiritual well-being in the event they use any of the information in this book for themselves, which is their constitutional right. The author and the publisher assume no responsibility for their actions.

Cover design by Frank Salazar.

Published 2014 by BookCrafters, Parker, Colorado.
BookCrafters@comcast.net
www.bookcrafters.net

Copies of this book may be ordered from
www.bookcrafters.net
and other online bookstores.

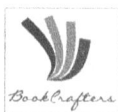

Foreword

The idea of the book was prompted after I was the receiving Hospice Nurse of Baby O when he passed away. The death of a child profoundly touched me in ways that changed my life forever. My outlook on life took a turn for the better. I became more insightful and aware of my life destiny. I was chosen by Hospice to deepen my awareness of my path thus far. Life was laced with death and grieving as a young child and throughout my life. I feel I have a very deep understanding of what people losing a loved one go through. I am not fearful of death.

This book further came into fruition when I injured my knee one week before going on a Canadian ski adventure with my partner. Being a lover of life, I decided I was going along anyway. I had a goal in mind; I had to finish this book while I was immobile. I could not change the things that already occurred. I had to have an open mind and stay busy with other things. A recurring theme was what to do when people pass. Death, a taboo subject. We talk about birth a lot easier. People are confused and don't know what to expect or how to be a caregiver. Hopefully this will give you some answers as a patient and a caregiver.

Disclaimer

This book is designed to provide information and motivation to our readers. It is sold with the understanding that the publisher is not engaged to render any type of psychological, legal, or any other kind of professional advice. The content of each article is the sole expression and opinion of the author, and not necessarily that of the publisher. The characters are fictitious even though they may seem like people you may know.

No warranties or guarantees are expressed or implied by the publisher's choice to include any of the content in this volume. Neither the publisher nor the individual author(s) shall be liable for any physical, psychological, emotional, financial, or commercial damages, including, but not limited to, special, incidental, consequential or other damages. Our views and rights are the same: you are responsible for your own choices, actions, and results.

Dedicated to my children,
Gavin and Mara Millette.

I will always love you!

Acknowledgements

I want to thank all the people that helped me along the way including my life partner, Matthew Kamper, my friends Valerie Latanzi, Inge Verhaegen, Teresa Cierco, Ellen Miller, Dudley Duel Underdahl, Tom Donohue, Michele Hudson Rothe, my siblings Inneke Debie, Baldwin Debie, Kristof Debie, my in-laws Bob Millette, Maggie Pederson, my kids Gavin Millette and Mara Millette, my Hospice patients and families, my instructor Connie Selzer, Mickey Krupa who we lost at age 42 due to a rare spinal cancer and so many more. Thank you all for being such an integral part in my life. I am forever grateful and indebted to you for your beauty and wisdom.

CONTENTS

How to embrace resilience.
Change, ready for the universe to unveil.
In the universe there is no success or failure
only the present moment.
The gift resides in every moment.

— Deepak Chopra

A new beginning
1979 in a small town outside of Brussels

I found myself alone wandering the small alleys around the church square, listening to the gossip of the elders and smelling fresh baked apple pies lingering, touching the green shutters and white painted brick walls of century old row houses. I was new to this town, did not know anybody. Mom and Dad decided to divorce which meant we were uprooted to Mom's birth town, Mollem. She inherited an 1880 duplex from an uncle who had just passed. I was the oldest of three, always expected to take care of everything and to be strong. I was eight years old, my brother five, and my sister new born.

Mom found a foreign letter in Dad's man-purse, the kind with red, blue and white vertical stripes on the edge and a big stamp " Par Avion." That was the end of their relationship; they had been high school sweethearts and conceived me in their senior year. They plotted to leave their Catholic strict homes. Life was shaky, Dad trying to finish school while Mom took care of us all at home.

My fondest memories where those of my amazing grandparents Pierre and Anna. Grandpa found Grandma in Germany while serving for the army during the Second World War. Grandma had a peculiar language of her own; it was neither German nor Flemish but a bastardization of both. Dad and Uncle even had Grandma's lingo down. They had a joie de vivre unlike anything I had experienced. Now I understand that this love of life may be of all their negative experiences they experienced. Grandpa lost an eye in the war and was thrown in jail for collaborating with the Germans. Grandma, on her death bed in 2001, kept telling me, "They are going to get me." "Who, Grandma?" I softly asked. Her eyes were full of fear, reliving the moments as an adolescent during the Hitler era. Grandma's family housed Jewish people in the cellar of their farm and fed them fresh eggs and bread and butter, kept them warm and alive, away from the Nazi's. Her entire life she lived with that fear, but it was unbeknownst to our family until her final day when she could not keep it a secret any longer.

I had no idea what I wanted to be when I grew up. I wanted to be like my grandparents, full of life and wonder. I played doctor and nurse in the playroom of my friend's converted attic. But didn't everybody play that? The curiosity of a young teenage girl and her male friends. Of course everything was benign with my plastic medical box filled with syringes, a stethoscope, some tongue depressors and a thermometer. I pretended to be Edith Cavell or Clara Barton with my white cap and Red Cross plastered on top.

Life went on in rural Belgium with many ups and downs as expected. Grandpa's life was tragically taken at age 62, and Grandma survived the gruesome accident. Grandpa bled to death in the arms of a policeman that unfaithful dreary December night at the crossroad of Linden straat en Molen beek. It was two a.m. and Grandpa had returned from their weekly band assembly, Grandpa played the trombone in a band of about 20 middle age musicians. They played Bach, Mozart, Vivaldi and other noteworthy pieces. I loved assisting them and reveling in the attention of all their friends. It was a social event with food and music galore.

That evening, I could not come; I was down with the stomach flu. Mom and Dad did not know how to deliver the news the next day and kept it silenced for a few days. I am sure they were talking amongst themselves on how to deliver the news to us three. Days later they sat my brother and me down, our sister was too young and would not understand. With an awkward pause, Mom said something terrible had happened and Grandma and Grandpa's car was hit by a drunk driver at 200km/hr. He did not stop at the crossroads and hit my cautious Grandpa who always stood at the crossroad looking right, looking left, and looking right again and again left. I could just imagine him standing at the crossroads being uber cautious and Grandma assisting him. I was numb and in denial, not my amazing grandparents. Grandma survived but she was in a coma.

Since I was the oldest of us three, I mustered up the courage and decided I wanted to see my grandma. I approached the elevator of St Donatus Hospital. Cautiously pressed number seven, the ride seemed to be forever. I stood there unraveling my scarf with Aunt Chris beside me trying to comfort me with her soft voice. The elevator stopped with an abrupt halt and a loud ding. I proceeded to the right stopping at the nurses' station, a young lady dressed in pure white dress and cap assisted me to room 705 and told me Grandma was still in a coma but can hear me. I peeked around the corner of the heavy wooden door and in the corner of the room was my grandma her hair long and flowing hooked up to tubes and vents and loud machines. Grandma had significant internal issues I was told and they had to put her in an induced coma. I did not know much about collapsed lungs, severed nerves around the eye, or broken limbs and ribs. She did not look like my grandma, I whispered, "I love you" with the hopes she would hear me, no twitch or jerk or slight movement was observed. I tried

3

to stay with Grandma stroking her hair now long and messy, touching her feet and arm tenderly.

Grandma came back to life six months later. It was summer time and school just finished and I had lots of time to spend with her. I would ride my old fashioned, no gear, back-brake bicycle from our town through country roads, small hills and cobblestone squares. I loved making the one hour trip through five towns to see my beloved grandma. We had tea time and lunches that lasted hours. I even spent some nights with her. We reminisced about life, read gossip magazines, watched gossip shows or the Euro song Festival. I even snuck out to the cemetery to say hi to Grandpa and told him everything was going fine out here.

I did not realize the connection I had with my grandparents, especially my grandma, till about a decade later. Already living in the United States with two kids of my own, I woke up in the middle of the night with visions of Grandma. I had the sudden urge to buy a ticket home for no apparent reason. Just like a mother knowing when her baby would be born, except I did not know why I was going home. I felt depressed for weeks. Doctors would say you have allergies. I had never had allergies in my life. Why now? I went with my gut and flew to Belgium without kids for a quick one week visit, only to find my grandma teetering at the edge of life, in and out of consciousness. Nurses would bring her morphine every few hours. The said it helped with oxygen delivery at the end of life. She appeared peaceful, taking shallow, fast breaths. I spend day and night with Grandma, singing songs she sang to me.

Hoppe, hoppe Reiter
wenn er fällt, dann schreit er
hoppe, hoppe Reiter
wenn er fällt, dann schreit er
fällt er in den Sumpf
macht der Reiter plumps

Hoppe, hoppe Reiter
wenn er fällt, dann schreit er
fällt er auf die Steine
tun ihm weh die Beine
fällt er in den Sumpf
macht der Reiter plumps

Hoppe, hoppe Reiter
wenn er fällt, dann schreit er
fällt er in den Graben
fressen ihn die Raben
fällt er in den Sumpf
macht der Reiter plumps?

— Ernst Wolf

Grandma took her last breath in my presence and I am glad I listened to the urge within me to see her one last time. Could she have been unconsciously calling me to say goodbye?

5

I have to go

The time had come that I had to leave. I had graduated high school in 1989 and wasn't sure about what to study not unlike many students my age. Dad signed me up at VLEKHO, specializing in languages because I excelled in that area. I lasted six months and knew school wasn't for me at the time. I found an au pair agency at the American Embassy in Brussels. I started the lengthy process of application papers and interviews. I was initially placed in Lubbock, Texas.

Ten days before my departure I was placed in Breckenridge, Colorado with a family of three kids, Rachel and Nathan, three year old twins, and Nichole, the oldest, a mature six year old. I prepared myself for the new venture; I only had a week and a half. I packed my Luis Vuitton suitcase to the gills with books, my favorite perfume, my ski boots and ski suit with outdated lime green gators, neon yellow zinc for high altitude sun protection.

March 19, 1991

I said my goodbyes to the family, my siblings, my aunt and uncle, cousins, Mom and Dad, my boyfriend, friends, Grandparents and my beloved dog Belle. They were excited for me but scared at the same time. At Zaventem, I checked in my suitcases, gave my parents and my siblings one last hug and disappeared behind the thick glass door. I looked back trying to get one last glimpse from my family but I could not locate them. They were swallowed by the crowds saying goodbye to their loved ones. It took six some hours to get to La Guardia Airport. I was ecstatic to catch the next plane from New York to Denver. Besides me in row 35, was a friendly middle aged man. He introduced himself as Michael.

"What's your name?" he kindly asked.

"Bieke," I whispered.

"What are you doing in Denver?" he asked.

I said, "I will be a nanny in the mountains of Colorado for a years, and I am planning to see the entire US on my time off."

He busted out laughing and said, "Honey, I am 45 and still haven't seen the entire United States." I was embarrassed and curious.

I arrived in Denver, Colorado, the following day from when I started travelling in Europe. A thin blonde woman greeted me at the arrival area; she had a cardboard sign with "Welcome Bieke" decoratively designed. "I am Michele, your host mother, welcome." We loaded up the SUV with my two big suitcases. She said we should hurry and leave because there is a grand winter storm brewing. We had two more hours to drive to the house.

My eyes were filled with wonder and fatigue simultaneously. The entire I-70 corridor was full of excitement, a herd of buffalo appeared in the corner of my eye passing Evergreen, then there was Buffalo Bill's Grave, Georgetown with mining, the Eisenhower tunnel. Once we passed the tunnel it was a full on blizzard. Cars were stopped on the side of the road and 18-wheelers were jack-knifed not allowing us to pass. The snowbank on either side dwarfed the SUV. I skied in France, Italy and Austria growing up, but I had never seen anything like this. We arrived at the home four hours after our expected arrival. The kids greeted me in the doorway wearing cozy pajamas with footies, holding there blankets. I took three steps up the steps leading to the living area and had to gasp for air. I curled myself up in the fetal position trying to find air in my tiny body. The kids were amused by my strange sea-level antics. "I am OK, kids," I smiled. I had an amazing year meeting great people in the community and this was the start of a new endeavor.

Dharma is much more than one's career or focus of activity in life. Dharma is the unstoppable force of evolution in the cosmos that impels everything forward toward self-awareness. Everyone has a purpose or dharma. If we didn't, we wouldn't exist at all.

–Deepak Chopra

Don't want
to return home

It was very apparent on May 19, 1992 as I stepped off the plane that I had reluctantly boarded in Denver, Colorado. It was an ordinary, overcast, cloudy, rainy, depressing day in my own country. The country I was born in 19 years ago. How could it be so foreign to me?

Locals were speaking their native tongues amongst themselves in the baggage claim area of Brussels International Airport at Zaventem, eager to get back to their families, friends, but mostly the country they love. As I pushed the small baggage cart intended for two small pieces of luggage. I carefully navigated the cart overloaded with trinkets from my travels abroad. Indian medicine bags, carefully crafted by the Hopi elder I met in Canyon De Chelley. Rocks from my hikes in the mountains of Colorado and the canyons of Utah and Arizona – rocks in all kinds of shapes, colors and sizes, some dull some sparkly. Sand from the desert outside of Moab, that I had collected consciously to show Mr. Goosens, my high school geology teacher back home. He was the teacher who was such an inspiration to me during my rough and tough high school years.

"Pardon, Madame, Excuse moi,"… I was pushed by a well-dressed, overweight, cigarette smoking, French speaking native, and I soon realized this was not home anymore. I understood all my native languages; I no longer understood their mannerisms, their actions. I should have been happy to be home.

"Next!" the border patrol belted out, as if I were deaf. I am a bit jet lagged and tired but I can hear you fine, sir, I thought to myself. Chin almost touching his high desk, eyes peaking over jet black, thick framed glasses, he abruptly asked, "Passport please," from inside his tiny glass cage. "Oh, you are a native, French or Flemish?" I wanted to tell him but I couldn't, he wouldn't care anyway. If I could, I would have told him that I'd just left my "real home," and now I have returned after my one year hiatus in the United States of America. He was just doing his job. "Next!" he screeched to the person in line.

My siblings and parents were jumping up and down behind the barrier outside the glass sliding door, visibly excited to see me, their oldest sister and daughter. I was happy to see them, although a bit groggy from my 12-hour flight, and excited they still looked the same. I had only been gone one year; to them it seemed like a decade.

"Wow, Sissy, your hair is so long and you are really tanned," my brother welcomed me.

My sister chimed in, "You gained a few pounds, must be all that good American processed food."

Most of all, my mother noticed I had a glow about me, and somehow she knew her oldest daughter would not stay long. "You look so calm and happy," she softly whispered. A mother's intuition is always right.

Once I passed the horrible feeling of jet lag and the longing for the people I met on my journey, I started calling travel agencies to book my trip back home; to the opportunities, friends and nature – back to the woman I was intended to be.

Graduation, Glenwood Springs,

May 5, 2012

Finally, graduation. I started this journey in the spring of 2002. Freshly divorced with two small children, I enrolled myself at the local college in a semester long EMT course. I enjoyed the medical field tremendously. It was new to me and exhilarating. My longtime friend got my foot in the door at the local hospital. She was a pharmacist at that location. I started night shifts on the floor as an EMT/ Caretech, meaning I assisted nurses taking vital signs, helping with ADL's (activities of daily living) such as showers, bed baths, transfers, ambulating and so on. It was a tough job and did it for 10 years while I was taking courses to get ready for nursing school. I loved the patient care and especially enjoyed the elder or very young. I received my acceptance letter to Colorado Mountain College in March of 2009. I pondered whether to accept it or not. I was never one to like school. I started nursing school the fall of 2009. It was the hardest thing I had ever done, being a single mom, working part-time and going to school full-time while driving one hour each way and sometimes three hours to perform clinicals.

As I sat there in my turquoise cap and gown ready to

claim the degree I so much wanted a decade ago. I was grateful for all the people who supported me in my journey, especially my kids who had seen me suffer. I glanced over to the right and spotted them in the sea of well-groomed folks holding colorful flowers. I could feel their joy for their mom who was now a Registered Nurse. I shed a tear for all the sacrifices made and another tear for the joy to come.

Then perhaps another hurdle to overcome as I prepared for the dreaded NCLEX, the State Exam all nurses have to take before being able to practice as a nurse. Months of preparatory work doing online tests and exercises to make you aware of the NCLEX way. A way that is a little peculiar to the average person, as a lot of these answers are not correct in a real life setting. On July 2nd I took my Board Exam in a commercial building in South Denver, Colorado. I was nervous; I left all my belongings at the front desk where the attendant gave me a locker key. She rambled off a plethora of rules and all I understood was, "You are not allowed to take anything inside."

I proceeded to the video screened area and took a seat in the small cubicle; there were three other students taking the exam. I was reminded I had six hours to complete the exam. I was ready to be done without having started yet. I anxiously hit the start button on the small screen. Being easily distracted, I slipped the thick black earphones over my head and adjusted them to fit. Questions 1, 2, 3, 4. I could not focus with those headphones any longer. I could hear the thumping and pulsating of my heart in my ears. I gathered my focus and two hours later the computer shut off. Panic set in, I wondered if I passed or failed. No way of knowing until I got the letter in the mail unless I did the self-test online on the Pearson View site.

I attempted to proceed with the test and I could not retest on Pearson View which could tell me I passed. Not completely certain, I paid the extra $7.95 to find out my results. Drum roll: from the pay site I was transferred to the Pearson View test results. In big bold letters it said, **You Passed**. That was all I needed to know.

I had heard horror stories of students not passing the Board Exam three times in a row and were suspended for a year. You may think, they should not be nurses. I disagree some of us are just not great test takers. The good news in my case is I will never have to take the dreaded NCLEX again unless I let my license lap. That is a relief in itself, to be done with studying for a little while.

I was lucky to have been chosen by a local Home Health and Hospice organization in my rural area. I had sent around 60 resumes to hospitals within a two-hour radius. No luck in this rural area. I received a text in September from the department I had worked in for a decade saying, "Dear Bieke, we have to let you go because you are over qualified in your current EMT position. I hope you understand." I was furious, ten years of my time and I am now overqualified? How about we will train you as a nurse and would love to keep you?

I started my job as a nurse at my current location and realized I really did not know anything after a decade of working with patients and a decade of school. The staff trained me for a month, I followed the other two nurses around soaking up all the information I could, reading up on conditions I had never heard of. They were understaffed, and sooner than expected, I was sent out on my own. I started July 28th and on August 6th I was assigned a Hospice patient with CHF-Congestive Heart Failure.

Every week I went out on a visit while he was stable; I shook in my boots for the first few weeks. All by myself, no other nurses or doctors to rely on. I was my own show, the phlebotomist, critical thinker, family counselor, ear nose and throat lady, you name it. I was alone out in the field with the nearest neighbor 10 miles away and no cell service.

One Tuesday afternoon Archie didn't seemed his usual self, he was tired, slumped over in his chair, pale and short of breath. A heart rate of 32 is not normal. It quickly dawned on me his pacemaker was failing. He was 95 years old and did not want another operation to replace the batteries. I had to keep him comfortable until he took his last breath which could be in an hour, a day or a week.

He had been asking me, "What am I doing here? Can I leave and be with my wife?" A question I could not answer. There is a time to be born and a time to leave this earth was my natural though, but I kept quiet, touched his veiny hands and listened to him.

And so my journey started in palliative and Hospice care as a newly graduated nurse. I had known the family for more than a decade and it was very difficult for me to care for him, not because of him, but them. Mostly because we had more than a nurse-patient relationship, we were like family and boundaries could not be reestablished. Or should I say, I failed to create boundaries.

The day I realized I could not safely care for this family was the day I was celebrating my son's birthday at a hut trip without cell service. I had left a generic message on my cell phone stating, "I am currently out of town and cell service, please call the office at (***-***-****), thanks for your call and have a great day!"

Once back in cell service on my way home, I received several messages. "Hi Bieke, this is Cara. Archie had another fall and has skin tears from his elbow to his wrist. Can you come have a look at this? I need your help."

I called her back, now three days later, to inquire if another nurse had looked at the wound and to see how Archie was. When she said no, I was furious and worried at the same time, worried about the liability of being a nurse, and furious because nothing was done. Archie now had a major infection and at 95 these don't heal easily.

That was the day I realized I had my hands full being a Hospice Nurse. I had no more privacy, was called at any hour of the day even though I never gave them my number. Patients like to stick with the same nurse especially at the end of life.

Archie passed away a month later at his home and is now united with his wife of 70 years. I enjoyed listening to his stories about the navy and his wife, they truly brought a smile to his face, and I am elated he is with Elle again looking down on me guiding me into the next adventure of Hospice nursing.

Hospice Experiences

Thanksgiving 2012

I have a lot to be grateful for: my health and my kids' health, a roof over our head and food to feed us. I got a call on my personal phone during our dinner. A worried voice on the other end utters in despair, "Bieke, it's Shirley. Sorry to bother you, I can't get ahold of anybody at the office. John is not doing well, can you come over?"

We had a policy at our office that we three nurses rotate call so our patients could call 24/7 and talk to a nurse. I couldn't get a call back from the nurse on call either, so I excused myself and proceeded to John's home. The bond you form with the patient's family is profound and it is almost that they want only you to give continuity of care. I completely sympathize with them. I love to stick with what is familiar too.

I arrived at half past eight to find John in distress. He was an educated 59 year old retired radiologist with lymphoma. He was sitting upright in bed with four pillows holding him, eyes wide open, breathing shallow fast breaths, and his mouth had a bluish tint around it. I ached for him and his family and humanly shed a tear in his presence. His very pregnant daughter was crying in the hallway, and his was wife by his side talking softly while holding his 200 pound, six foot frame whispering, "I love you."

By ten that night John was comfortable, and so was his family, and I returned to my home where my kids were patiently waiting for me. John lived another four days surrounded by his family and passed peacefully in the arms of his wife in the comfort of his home. I was called in at 5 a.m. to help Shirley care for Jon. She wanted to be there until the end.

He was one of the first deaths I assisted and was thoroughly shaken by the magnitude of death and grief taking me back to when my grandpa died. Grandpa was 62, taken too early from me, his 12 year old granddaughter. I had started dying myself at 12 and realized these experiences with Hospice care are bringing me back to 1983.

I had not faced my past, never talked about the grief I carried around. I trotted through life with a smile on my face, a façade, hiding the anger and sadness of a life taken too early. I was on stage, the heavy Burgundy velvet curtain had parted and I was wide open, naked to the audience. I would have bursts of crying while taking a walk in nature. There was no reason to cry but I allowed it, and I realized this was a natural progression of grieving that had been suppressed for twenty-some years. There was no more room for sadness, I hunger for freedom and to surrender to the beauty of life as it is. I had to choose life in the face of death.

My life started to change for the better once I realized my life purpose and why Hospice picked me. I have much gratitude for all the experiences I faced in my line of work.

Another day in the office

I clocked in at 7 a.m. to finish the mounds of paperwork associated with Medicare and Medicaid that had to be submitted within a short timeframe. Useless information that is repetitive and it is unknown who takes care of it after it gets submitted to the State. The Director and Manager usually clocked in at 10 a.m. I guess this was a perk to my Hospice RN job; I could do the paperwork at a time convenient to me. On the other hand, people tend to pass in the middle of the night. Many times I was woken at 2 a.m. by a family member telling me that their loved one had just passed or was about to pass.

The Director strolled in shortly after the Clinical Manager; she passed by my tiny cubicle as she does every morning. About 30 minutes later she approached me, looked over her thin pink reading glasses, and curiously asked, "Are you available to admit this 59 year old with prostate cancer?" I said, "Sure. Can I see his history and physical, and his address info?" I educated myself on his condition and phoned him to set up an appointment to admit him. We usually have to admit a patient the day after discharge from a hospital or the day after we get the referral from the physician.

"Hello, this is Bieke. I am a nurse with Hospice. How are you?"

An educated English woman's voice responded on the other end, "I am fine, and you?"

"Great," I replied. "Our office just received a referral from your husband's oncologist. What is a good time to come by and do a Home Evaluation and possible Hospice admit?"

"Can you come at one?" she asked.

I arrived at the home a few minutes early with my medical bag including an O2 saturation meter, blood pressure cuff and sphygmomanometer, a temporal thermometer, my stethoscope and the admit paperwork. Chloe welcomed me at the door and guided me upstairs where Mark was sitting in his chair looking rather pale and short of breath.

MP had been married to CP for 30 years, high school sweethearts. They had a daughter who was a senior in the local private high school. They were both high powered individuals, CEO's of companies with 250 employees.

He wasn't feeling well but pretended he was just fine. I could sense he would not be around a lot longer, but he was hanging on. He was diagnosed with prostate cancer about a year ago; unfortunately it was discovered too late and had spread to his liver and bones. He could either accept the losses graciously or live the remaining days in misery. I completed the whole body assessment and completed the paperwork for a Home Health admit.

MP was slumped over gasping for air in a tripod position. His sentences were short. I advised him to conserve his energy. MP had recently been released from the local hospital after a chest tube was placed to remove the extra fluid in his lungs. He was hanging on for his daughter Libby, who will soon be without her Dad. He wasn't ready to accept Hospice yet. Hospice was perceived as giving up.

Weekly visits were made to make sure his pain was controlled and he was comfortable. He denied needing Hospice care. I suggested a speech therapist for his difficulty of swallowing; even though I knew the cause was an increase of tumor growth making it difficult to swallow, it might give him a little relief.

The following week I received a call from his wife at 9 p.m. "Bieke, "she calmly uttered. "Can you come over? He is breathing funny. I don't know what to do." I was hanging vancomycin for another Home Health patient we had at the time of her call. I told her I should be there within the hour.

When I arrived, Patty, his oncologist, was present. MP had visibly started the active dying process. His eyes were looking upward, he was unconscious and his breathing was labored and rapid. His daughter lay curled up in the fetal position on her daddy's left side. She wasn't crying, she was silently 'being' with her daddy.

CP asked, "Is it appropriate to take him to the ER?" I took her to the dimly lit hallway and explained in a calm voice looking at her eyes, "Your husband is passing now; this could last from a few hours to a few days. We need to keep him comfortable. Tell him you love him and simply be with him." She stoically looked at me, and returned to the room. I administered 0.5 ml of liquid morphine in his cheek and asked CP if she needed anything else. She replied "No, I will call you. Thank you."

I returned home, went to sleep and at 11:15 at night I received a call that MP had passed. I went to the home and asked CP how much time she needed before the funeral home came to get the body of her husband. "You can call them now," she replied. I called the firefighters and the funeral home and assisted Libby and Mom with emotional support. I gave each them time to be with their beloved father and husband.

I removed the oxygen tubing from his nose. I washed the body with a lukewarm wash cloth and put him in a favorite outfit laid out by Libby. The firefighters arrived with a stretcher. MP was on the second floor, and we collectively waited for the funeral home folks to arrive. The mood was somber and quiet. CP was matter of fact and wanted to see her husband leave down the stairs, through the door and into the van. I asked gently, "Do you really want to watch?" She confidently replied, yes, without hesitation. She did not show any emotion at that time.

I stood next to her watching MP brought down on a stretcher by four strong firefighters. They came around the first set of stairs, and faced us standing by the landing. I looked over to CP and made sure she was coping and touched her tiny frame. She said goodbye to him after 35 years of being together. She had to let go and surrender. I hugged her when MP disappeared down the meandering driveway, while snowflakes melted on our warm faces, blending with tears of relief and sadness.

Baby O

Another sad day in our community, Baby O passed away last night. I unfortunately was on call. Patients seem to know when I am on call and I was dubbed "angel of death" by my coworkers.

Baby O was diagnosed with Zellweger's disease at one week of birth.. The prognosis is poor; most infants don't survive past six months of age. Zellweger's is a rare chromosomal disorder that only affects a small percentage of infants. Symptoms of these disorders include an enlarged liver; characteristic facial features, such as a high forehead, underdeveloped eyebrow ridges, and wide-set eyes; and neurological abnormalities such as mental retardation and seizures. Infants with Zellweger syndrome also lack muscle tone, sometimes to the point of being unable to move, and may not be able to suck or swallow. Some babies are born with glaucoma, retinal degeneration, and impaired hearing. Jaundice and gastrointestinal bleeding are common.

I first met baby O and his mom when he was two months old when I attended the fifth birthday party for her daughter. His regular nurse was not available; I had time and loved infants. I started the feeding pump, burped him and changed his diaper. He appeared to be like any other infant except for his clubbed feet and wide forehead. He cooed and made infant noises. I kept track of his seizures in a small pocket journal on the night table next to his crib. He had been seizing a handful of times a day. I enjoyed spending time with this little angel.

Moments with infants who have limited time are precious

and make me realize how truly fortunate I am to have two healthy children.

I received a call from Jennie, Baby O's mom, at four in the afternoon on Sunday. "Hi, this is Jennie. I have a question for you."

"OK, what is it?"

"Is it normal for Baby O to have a bloody diaper?"

I replied, "No, but I will check with your pediatrician. I will call you back as soon as I hear from him. Do you need me to come over?"

"No that is not necessary, thank you."

Baby O's feedings had been discontinued the day before due to his increased number of seizures and the family had decided to cease all life prolonging measures. A tough decision for parents to make; to let go of their sweet baby. At 9 p.m. I received a call. A calm voice on the other end informed me that baby O had passed away.

I gathered my coat and shoes and drove to their home in the quaint mining town. I was in anguish; I had dealt with many deaths but not a baby's death. I collected myself outside in the pebble-stone driveway. I had to be strong for them. It was serene; the snow was falling peacefully from the heavens and I could hear the angels sing. A snowshoe hare scurried in the bushes. I knocked three times on the red painted front door.

Jennie opened the door somewhat subdued. I hugged her which seemed like forever. "Come in, he is upstairs."

I asked the family what they needed at the time. "Can I wash him for you and dress him in a favorite outfit?"

"I don't know," she hesitated, "I have never dealt with this before."

"If you need more time alone with him let me know."

Special arrangements were made with the funeral home. The parents were to drive baby O themselves. I prepared baby O for departure. His sister was sleeping next door with Jennie's grandparents. How will she react tomorrow when she awakens? I am sad for her, I know grieving is a lifelong task and I prayed she has better resources than I did when I lost my grandpa. My heart aches for her, five years old and her baby brother is gone and did not come back and will never come back in this physical world.

Under the weeping willow tree,
I sit and ponder
I wonder what life will be without you.
I miss holding you
I miss the soft gurgling noises
I know you are with someone special
Holding you
With a touch of an angel
Love all around you and within you
Never experiencing hate or fear.
I will always love you
And never forget you.

— Gerlinde Debie-Millette

Alzheimer's

In December I meet Jeff and Charlotte, married for 50 years living in a small mountain community. Charlotte had Alzheimer's, rather progressive and had declined a lot in the past few months. Jeff did not know how to care for her as she now needed 24-hour supervision due to her mental status. I was assigned to them after Charlotte had a fall and needed a nurse and physical therapy to work with her. We were all worried about her safety.

Jeff and I talked about the possibility of looking into a nursing home or Alzheimer's Unit. He could not fathom having Charlotte, his bride of 50 years admitted, and continued to care for her, a full-time job which Jeff loved to do. The issue was they were in their 80s and the body naturally cannot keep up as it used to. Jeff had his own issues dealing with diabetes and heart failure. I visited them weekly for a month. Charlotte would recognize my colorful Keens' uniforms with patterns; she loved them.

I loved visiting with their family and Anna, the Mexican aid, who helped Jeff with laundry, cleaning, cooking and basic supervision of Charlotte. One morning at my regular 10 o'clock meeting, she seemed different. Jeff reported she had not gotten out of bed and was crying a lot more. She denied pain and just told me she is sad but could not tell me why. I consulted with Jeff on Hospice care. He could get more help, aides to wash her, volunteers to read to her and supervise her.

The problem was with the insurance regulations. In order to qualify for Hospice care, an individual has to have a life expectancy of six months or less and have a terminal diagnosis. Alzheimer's can drag on forever – decades, and in the grand scheme this would not be an option for her. I consulted with her Primary Care Physician, and she agreed we could start Charlotte on Hospice care. Worst case scenario we could discharge her before the six month period ended and transfer her care to Home Health or a Long Term Care Nursing facility.

Insurance providers want to see a decline in the patient's status in order to pay for the services. It broke my heart to see a couple, after all these years of marriage, in this state of dependence, and it pained me to hear the quiver in his voice every time I mentioned placement in a nursing home. He loved her the same way he loved her when they first met 65 years ago. What an inspiration in today's day and age. Truly touching.

There is no guarantee in life

For over a year I cared for Natalie, an educated woman, who was diagnosed with Bulbar ALS a few months before her 60th birthday. She lived with her husband, a Labrador, and a cat in a beautiful log home at the top of Windy Ridge. Two daughters lived outside the home. Her youngest daughter focused on caring for her mom full-time since Natalie's husband had a full-time job. Natalie regressed month after month with lots of hospitalizations concerning her lungs, mostly aspiration pneumonia and mucus plugs.

Amyotrophic Lateral Sclerosis is a progressive neurological disease that is fatal. Bulbar relates to the pons and medulla of the brainstem which controls the throat, tongue, jaw and face. When these motor neurons die the brain is unable to transmit instructions to the voluntary muscles.

Over the course of the year she lost her speech and relied heavily on Siri on her iPad. She would type in words and Siri would talk for her. Her respiratory was compromised and soon she needed to be placed on a ventilator and a feeding tube due to the inability to swallow or breathe on her own.

I loved visiting her, we had so much in common, and just being near her was therapeutic for both of us. With minimal communication we enjoyed each other's company. We talked about herbal remedies for minor bruises or abrasions. I made her a poultice with arnica and lavender for her sore muscles on her shoulder. I soaked a cheese cloth in mint herbal tea, pulverized the herbs with a garlic pestle and wrapped them in the cheese cloth with a few drops of lavender essential oil. We communicated by sign language and technology.

The last few days of her life, Natalie became more distant, her respirations were shallow and her pulse oximetry measured 81% on 5-liters of concentrated oxygen. She was sleeping more and not communicating at all. I received a call at 10 p.m. on a Thursday evening from Hank. He was concerned because her Foley catheter was not draining. It had just been placed a few days ago and the family thought perhaps it was not placed correctly. I went to the home with an irrigation kit, knowing this may not be the case; she was simply dying.

I spoke with all three daughters and Hank, and told them to prepare to say goodbye. I explained that at the end of life the kidneys, heart and vascular systems stop working and not a lot of urine is produced. They requested to have the irrigation done and I gladly did it. The Foley was draining sufficiently; a scant amount of dark brown urine was extracted.

Natalie was not conscious, I touched her hand which felt cold, and wished her a peaceful departure. Lulu the cat, curled up by her feet and Jasper, the dog, faithfully flanked her side as they knew she was standing in the middle of the tunnel, this time not turning back, but instead she was reaching for the light.

I stayed with the family for moral support, while happy

stories of their mom and wife were exchanged. Laughter and tears all together, a melody touched all. Natalie took her last breath surrounded by her entire close family. She was such an inspiration to me; she fought an amazing battle and did it with grace and poise.

Ann Marie

Meanwhile I was assigned to a case about an hour from my home base. Ann Marie was diagnosed with melanoma last year. A little spot was found by her hairdresser on her head. Exactly one year later the little black spot had engulfed her entire skull and bilateral ears, occluding her left eye. It was a smelly, thick black peeling scab about an inch thick. I did not know what to expect.

I knocked three times on the front door of this century old quaint periwinkle Victorian home with bright yellow accents on the window and door frames. Unanswered, I knocked a bit harder, and the dog began barking. One of the daughters welcomed me with open arms. Her sister and Jackie had been caring for their mom for a few weeks by themselves. They appeared exhausted and confused. She led me through a narrow hallway to a small back room flanked by angels and praying Mother Marys. Ann Marie lay motionless in her bed sideways with pillows under her hips and back. She had gone from an average 130 pound frame to perhaps 80 pounds, with bones protruding, making it painful to lie on her back.

I quietly introduced myself leaning towards her. I assessed her, and by the looks of her demeanor I felt she was close to death. She exhibited the signs of nearing death within a week. She slipped in and out of consciousness, was fatigued, not mobile, was sleeping a lot more and was talking to the deceased.

She was angry about dying and asked me if she could be revived once. I calmly explained that having a few broken ribs from being revived may not be fun to live with on top of the ailments of the cancer that had spread to her brain and bones. I assured it was her choice. She sighed and signed the DNR. The Do Not Resuscitate order is placed in sight of the emergency personnel, perhaps on the fridge, so they know not to perform CPR or resuscitate her. I felt her disappointment with my answer. She realized she was dying and nothing would bring her back. She looked at me with inquiring eyes and uttered a mumbled sentence, "Would you have undergone treatment that kills everything in your body?" I looked at her with a reassuring stare stating she made the right decision.

I excused myself to the back room with the daughters. They had many questions, "She hasn't been hungry, what can we feed her?" I calmly explained that this is one of the signs of nearing death. The older daughter started crying. I touched her shoulder gently; she knew her mom would not be around much longer. I plainly said, "The body is not hungry and is letting go. This can take a few days, to weeks. Listen to her, if she asks for something, prepare it for her."

Jackie felt inadequate, unable to keep her mother nourished. I assured her it is really OK to feel like this, allow it and focus on her needs the best you can. I left her a small handout, which you will find at the end of this book, about how to care for a dying patient. She thanked me and hugged me. As I walked out the door, I reminded both of them to call our on-call nurse number in case they have questions or they need a visit.

Two days later, on December 6th, a dark gloomy winter day, I was called to the home to facilitate Ann Marie's final moments. She was anxious, grasping for breath, moving side to side in her bed. Family members and Father Bob trickled into her room one by one to say goodbye to a soul taken too soon. There was crying, storytelling and reminiscing about a life well lived. I squeezed a few drops of Atropine in her cheek, to dry up the secretions that she could no longer swallow. The unsoundly rattle, often called the death rattle, was overbearing. Her companion Willie, the dog she adopted when her husband passed away seven years ago, was pacing back and forth from the bedroom to the kitchen. He was in tune with her and knew she was passing, not in distress, letting go and surrendering.

Can't let go

It was in the fall of 2013 that I was hired at a small rural hospital at 10,152 feet above sea level. It had an interesting population to say the least. Residents at the local nursing home were over 80 years old with the majority being in the mid-90's and one feisty lady was over 100 years old.

Alda caught my eye; she weighed 86 pounds fully clothed, bones protruding through her gown. She could not talking due to a previous brain injury, was bed-bound, and ate or drank minimally. She was a DNR, do not resuscitate, but we were keeping her alive with fluids and antibiotics and unnecessary treatments. This went on for months because the three siblings could not agree on her end of life care.

One daughter said, "Well, my brother can't let go."

"Has he visited lately?" I inquired caringly.

"No, he is too busy in Florida with work. But my other brother is on his way."

Charley said, "I don't want to put Mom down like a dog."

I found this to be a rather harsh statement. I gave him a booklet, "Gone from My Sight" by B Kearney, in the hopes that he would read it and have a better understanding of end of life care. Two siblings were on board with transitioning her to comfort care and stopping all life prolonging measures. But one was not, and that meant we had to keep going. Every morning I wondered if she was gone. For months I saw her regress, but with all the medical advances, we were keeping her alive.

Alda had opened my eyes to being mindful of my wishes for my end of life. Advanced Directives or a living will should be drafted now so my kids won't keep me alive when there are certain decisions I won't be able to make due to unforeseen circumstances.

On April 9th Alda celebrated another birthday. She was still waiting for her son to visit from Florida and hanging on by a thread. She lay motionless in the hospital bed taking fast shallow breaths, slipping in and out of consciousness. I had visions of my grandma waiting for me to arrive to say her last goodbye. I softly whispered to Alda touching her boney hand, "It's OK, you can go, everything will be all right."

And then there was Frankie

Frankie was diagnosed with Spinal Muscular Atrophy Type Two, a genetic disorder that affects the control of muscle movement, when he was six months old. It is caused by a loss of specialized nerve cells, called motor neurons, in the spinal cord and the part of the brain that is connected to the spinal cord. The loss of motor neurons leads to weakness and wasting of muscles used for activities such as crawling, walking, sitting up, and controlling head movement.

In Frankie's case, his breathing and swallowing was affected. Multiple tests confirmed the diagnosis. At age six he was placed on a ventilator and a gastronomy tube was inserted due to his inability to eat safely.

I had the pleasure of meeting him when I needed to pick up extra shifts to supplement my Hospice salary. Every

Sunday night I would leave home at 8 p.m. and drove over Battle Mountain and Tennessee Pass to reach his home in Leadville Colorado at 10,200 feet. On a good night, without snow or ice, it took me an hour.

I loved spending time with him; he was such a genuine, true and honest person who never ever complained He was one of those rare people that make you appreciate your life the way it is. These are the cards he was dealt and he was going to play them well.

I arrived at his home around 10 p.m. to find him on the phone talking to his girlfriend who lives in Texas. A normal conversation between lovers. He talked about the day, about his music and activity but most of all he told her he loved her. I tried to give them privacy while I was checking the ventilator settings and getting all the supplies ready. When he finished his conversation, I returned the phone to the recharger and got his treatments ready.

"How is it going today? Did you have a good day?" I inquired.

"Yes, I worked on my music" his soft voice replied. "You want to hear it?" he eagerly asked.

"Of course" I said. He loved writing and composing rap music and had a close connection with a rapper in LA. The music was deep and true to his state, but it was an outlet for him.

"Are you ready for the albuterol treatment?" He nodded in agreement. We joked and laughed. He had such a great sense of humor and positive outlook.

Frankie was 28 with two college degrees, a very intelligent human being with physical limitations; he did not want this genetic disease to be his identity. He was wheelchair bound and dependent on the ventilator and a feeding tube. That was the way it was, nothing could be changed. He accepted his condition and lived his life to the best of his ability. I

34

touched his deformed hands and massaged them gently with the touch of an angel.

He wanted to learn Flemish; we started with numbers and then simple words. He loved the challenge of learning a new language.

I lay his contractured frame in bed on his right side and tuck him in. His legs are always at a 90 degree angle, his wrists bent at a slight angle inward. I softly whispered, "Don't let the bed bugs bite." Throughout the night he asked to be turned from side to side. He was completely dependent on me for movement. Frankie had a Home Health Nurse for eight hours in the daytime and eight hours per night, four nights a week. His mom works as a Certified Nurse Assistant four days a week, and that schedule allowed her to get a good night's sleep so she could be productive. She loved her son and Frankie loved her.

*When you are joyous, look deep into your heart
and you shall find it is only that which has
given you sorrow that is giving you joy.*

-Kahlil Gibran, the Prophet

A few facts
we know about death

1. There is no possible way to escape death. No-one ever has, not even Jesus, Buddha, or other well known. Of the current world population of over six billion people, almost none will be live a 100 years except for those few exceptions, like my 106 year old patient.
2. Life has a definite, inflexible limit and each moment brings us closer to the finality of this life. We are dying from the moment we are born.
3. Death comes in a moment and its time is unexpected. All that separates us from the next life is one breath.
4. The duration of our lifespan is uncertain. The young can die before the old, the healthy before the sick.
5. The weakness and fragility of one's physical body contribute to life's uncertainty.
6. The body can be easily destroyed by disease or accident, for example cancer, AIDS, vehicle accidents, or other disasters.
7. Worldly possessions such as wealth, position, money can't help.
8. Relatives and friends can neither prevent death nor go with us.
9. Even our own precious body is of no help to us. We have to leave it behind like a shell, an empty husk, an overcoat.

Caring at the end of life

Listen and be present

Society does not know much about death. Death is portrayed peacefully in the movies with a person taking their last breath in a sterile setting. I have only witnessed a handful of peaceful deaths and mostly they were the elderly in their 90s. My role as a Hospice Nurse is to give emotional support and direction to the family and patient. As you consider providing care and support to the terminally ill patient, it is important to stop and take personal inventory of your own fears, and experiences with dying. Most people can remember their first experience with a dying person. It may have been a loved one or someone you have cared for. You may have had the experience of a sudden and tragic death of a friend or loved one. If you have never experienced the death of a loved one, you may fear caring for someone you love and care for. For example, you may have elderly parents and even though you know death is inevitable, you may have fears concerning their deaths.

Our first experiences with death frame our feelings and thought processes. They can add to or alleviate our fears. It is helpful to the patient and family if caregivers provide a sense of calmness and assurance in the face of death. This stresses the importance of dealing with individual anxieties and fears prior to caring for the terminally ill patient.

One step toward understanding our fears is to look at misconceptions about dying. Misunderstandings or myths about dying may exist and can interfere with people receiving the best possible care at the end of their life. For example, you may fear that patients will hallucinate and seizure sometime before death. You may worry that pain won't be controlled or treated to the level you want for your patient.

Take a moment to reflect on the losses in your life. Losses may include the death of a loved one, friend, or a public figure. Losses may also involve the death of a beloved pet or loss of a home or other important possessions. Your reaction to loss may depend on the stage of your life and the intensity of the relationship. You may not realize that you have been grieving since the divorce of your parents long ago due to losing your childhood.

Ways of being "present" include:

- Sit in comfortable silence.
- Listen attentively.
- Participate in conversation as the patient wishes.
- Gently touch the patient as appropriate.
- Read to the patient.
- Pray with the patient.
- Reminisce with the patient, valuing their life and experiences.
- Recognize the time for the patient's rest.
- Identify other means of letting the patient know his or her life is valued and that spending time with him or her is still important to you.

During this time of personal crisis, it is important to be present with the patient and family while demonstrating patience and compassion as they travel through a myriad of emotions and questions.

Anticipating the needs of the patient and family may require practice. Asking leading questions, open-ended questions requiring more than a "yes" or "no" answer, is one method of communication that allows for and encourages freedom of expression.

How can I best support you?
What can I do that would be most helpful for you today?
What is most troublesome to you?
What information can I attempt to clarify for you?

The family may not want to ask questions about the condition of their relative in front of him or her. Identify these communication needs and develop a plan of care that will meet the patient and family. Family conferences are often effective in bridging the communication gaps and misunderstandings between family members and the patient. The strength of a health care team is for members to share their observations to better assess communication needs and develop measures to meet them.

Since anxiety is often inevitable during the dying process, it is necessary for the professional to assess the reason behind the anxiety in order to address it. Anxiety may be related to spiritual, financial, emotional, relational, physical, or other concerns. However, it is difficult to treat anxiety without adequate communication.

It is important to recognize that each patient may have anxieties that may change from day to day or from one visit to another. Since the patient has not traveled this journey before, many patients have questions and fears. They may fear the process of dying more than death itself. For example, they may fear loss of bowel and bladder control or they may be concerned that they will experience severe pain during the dying process.

Support and education is often concentrated on the family and other caregivers who are coping with the anticipated loss of their loved one. We want to teach them how to care for their loved one's physical and emotional needs. However, it is imperative that the needs of the patient are not overlooked since the patient faces the loss of "everyone" and "everything" familiar to them. Adequate time and appropriate methods of communication should be considered a priority in the assessment of anxiety and related symptoms as it relates to both to the patient and to the family.

Anxiety may be a result of the dying process with underlying physical causes such as an increase in pain, respiratory distress, need for a change in position, a distended or full bladder, constipation, or other physical reasons. Use of pharmacological interventions such as Ativan, low dose morphine, or in more severe cases, Haloperidol, may provide temporary, intermittent, or long-term relief. The use of anti-cholinergic Atropine drops to dry up secretions, Tylenol suppositories to break a fever is helpful. Complimentary modalities such as relaxation therapy, massage, music and imagery may provide temporary or permanent relief. The team of professionals is integral to the assessment and treatment of anxiety, facilitating peace, and promoting a level of acceptance for the patient.

What to do when the patient is sleeping more:

- During the time they are awake be attentive to their needs and tell them you love them.
- Get sleep when they sleep and ask for a back-up to relieve you through the night.
- Speak in a soft voice. Don't assume that the patient can't hear you because they appear to be sleeping.
- Have a care journal and a list of back-up help. You can organize tasks for them so you don't experience burn out.

What to do when patient withdraws:

- Realize that they are going inward to work on the heart and spirit.
- Say what needs to be said, if appropriate, like goodbye and I love you.
- Realize this is not a time of rejection for you.
- Talk to friends and family. This time may be very emotional.

What to do when the patient gets weak:

- Provide a safe environment. Remove rugs that may be a tripping hazard, provide a call bell (Cow bell, tambourine, container with empty pistachio shells).
- Provide the patient with a walker, cane, wheelchair, commode, shower bench. These items can be provided by the Salvation Army or senior center on a loan basis. If not available, an order can be obtained from your doctor and these items can be purchased.
- Respect their independence and privacy.
- Consider having a Certified Nurse Assistant help a few times per week.
- Have direct communication with the patient.

What to do when the patient is afraid:

- Watch for signs of restlessness and/or crying.
- Open communication. What are you afraid off? Are you in pain?
- Continue laughing and living.
- Tell them you are there for them. You are not alone. Continue touching and talk to them softly.
- Have soothing music in the background playing softly.
- Ask them what they are afraid of. Pain, being alone, death, doubt about the way they lived their life, leaving things undone, loss of control?

As a caregiver you can watch for signs of restlessness and anxiety. You can listen with an open mind to what they have to say. Remind them you are there for them. For many people the end of life means looking back at a life lived. Working through disappointments, failures and negative parts of the journey may cause more anxiety. Seeking forgiveness and love become basic lessons to let go.

What to do when the patient is in pain:

- Keep a medication journal.
- Obtain a different dose or brand of pain medication from your doctor.
- Use massage, music or diversional modalities.
- Use a mantra.

What to do when the patient loses appetite:

- Don't force feed; this is a normal finding at the end of life. Foods don't taste good and it takes a tremendous amount of energy to digest foods.
- Ask the patient what sounds good like pudding, ice cream, smoothie, their favorite food. Listen to them.
- Provide small sips of water or ice chips.
- Moisten the lips with water based moisturizer.
- Provide constant mouth care with toothbrush or swabs.

What to do when the patient becomes confused:

- Speak to them in a calm voice. Introduce yourself.
- Provide around the clock supervision.
- Get back up help.
- Tell them you are there for them.

What to do when bowel and bladder function changes:

- Provide dignity and respect.
- Pain meds cause constipation, make sure to take a daily laxative. If still eating provide fiber in the diet.
- You may want to have a Foley catheter placed, use of protective pants and pads.
- Have wet wipes available for easy clean up and room deodorizer.
- Have a daily care system available, cleaning the area and applying a zinc barrier cream.

Preventing skin breakdown:

- Turn the person every two waking hours, propping pillows behind the back, knees, ankles.
- Keep the skin clean and dry.
- Don't massage or rub reddened areas.
- Depending on the degree of skin breakdown, there are specialized treatments your doctor can prescribe to alleviate pain and further damage.

What to do when a fever strikes:

- Provide a moist towel and place on neck, armpits or forehead.
- Change clothing and linens often to promote a dry environment.
- Medications to lower a fever. Tylenol suppositories are effective.
- Don't bathe in cold water.

What to do when breathing changes:

Sometimes the breathing may sound like gurgling or rattling. This is usually a late sign and may be evident when the person cannot clear his throat any longer on his own due to the reflex not working. They are not suffering or drowning. The person is most likely unconscious at this time and not aware. The pattern of breathing may be irregular.

- You can put pillows behind the persons back or if you have a hospital bed raise the head of the bed. They may want to sit up in a chair.
- With swabs or a moist cloth clear secretions from the mouth.

- Apply a few Atropine drops in the mouth to dry up secretions.
- Turn the person to the side.

Difficulty swallowing:

As the body weakens it becomes much harder to swallow. This may lead to choking or aspiration pneumonia.

- Instead offer ice chips, cold washcloths soaked in water to moisten the mouth.
- Provide mouth care every two hours while awake.
- Apply a water based moisturizer for the lips
- You may want to talk to your healthcare provider about obtaining liquid forms of medications versus pills.

Near death awareness:

- They seem confused and disoriented.
- They have conversations with the already deceased.
- May talk about bright lights and objects not visible to you.
- Make hand gestures and swat at air.
- Will talk about dying.

This may be symbolic to them. They are ready to transition and are asking you permission, forgiveness and they are actually saying goodbye.

You can help them by:

- Listening, not correcting them.
- Being with them fully. Being present.
- Ask who they see and how they make them feel.

At the time of death:

- Breathing stops.
- Bowel and bladder function may be lost.
- The mouth is open.
- Eyes don't blink and pupils are large.
- No pulse or heartbeat.

May I be filled with loving kindness.
May I be well.
May I be peaceful and at ease.
May I be happy.

— Dalai Lama

Useful tips for Caregivers

According to the Webster dictionary a caregiver is a person who gives help and protection to someone (such as a child, an old person, or someone who is sick).

Caregiving is a big task including many jobs that may change over the progression of the disease. You may find yourself cooking, cleaning, picking up medications, being a chauffeur to doctor appointments, listener, reader, and delegator. The key is not to get burned out. I have seen many caregivers at the end of their rope and are unable to care for the individual. I recommend getting other family members involved, friends, members of the community, a Hospice team if applicable. Having a support network is paramount. Who makes you laugh when you are down? What and who is important to you? You need a solid support crew.

Some tips from other caregivers:

1. When preparing meals, prepare large quantities so you can freeze them for a future date.
2. Start a care journal.
3. Assign one member of the family to give updates by email, phone or special care website.

4. Screen your calls; let the answering service pick up the calls. Hang a "Do not disturb sign." On the door.
5. Minimize grocery trips by buying in bulk especially TP, Laundry detergent, rice, pasta, cereals.

When people offer to help don't hesitate to give them a task, whether it is going to the post office, the grocery store, or hardware store. Be prepared to delegate.

Caregiving is a challenging job just performing the tasks listed above. In reality it is about relationships, the worries and changes, dreams and disappointments. Caring for someone with a life limiting illness is an up and down roller coaster with many moments of changes, losses and grieving. Grieving does not occur when someone passes. It starts before, you as the caregiver may be grieving about change in relationship, loss of activity, loss of freedom, wondering what the future holds.

Over the years, caregivers have taught us that caring for a terminally ill individual is a life changing experience. In the midst of hurt and sadness, we grow and learn and become a better person. As a nurse for terminally ill patients I have definitely grown into the person I wanted to be. So many have taught me invaluable life lessons and even though it was not the avenue I wanted to take graduating Nursing School, this path helped me grow. Hospice care picked me because that is what I needed at that time in my life. I am grateful and filled with love for the families and patients touching my life with grace and wisdom.

Focusing on lessons learned and being grateful can shift your attention from the difficulties to the rewards.

Try asking yourself the following questions:

Why did I choose to care for _____?

Through caregiving I have learned._____

What am I grateful for?_____

In what ways have I surprised myself caring for_____?

What to expect at the end of life

Death is unpredictable, it can come suddenly, but more often it comes after a long illness where we see a gradual decline of physical and mental systems. For some this may take hours, days, weeks or months. Every experience is unique. You may notice more drowsiness and sleepiness, withdrawal from the world, increased weakness.

One month before death

The patient may sleep most of the time. However, the patient may awaken, particularly when a new person or non-family member attempts conversation. This can be disturbing to the family who has tried in vain to converse with the patient who has shown little response. Explain to the family that the patient's response to a stranger is thought to be due to an unfamiliar voice causing a startling response.

Other behavior that may be observed in the final weeks of life is the patient picking at his or her clothes and increased agitation. He or she may also seem to lose their grounding on this earth and may appear to be in two worlds. The patient may enter into a conversation for a short time, and then drift out to a semi-conscious state.

They may mouth words that are unintelligible, or call out names of deceased loved ones. The patient can often be brought back to the current world with conversation or with physical stimulation such as repositioning.

Physical changes at this time may include the following:

- Loss of bodily functions such as incontinence of urine and/or stool
- Decreased pulse rate and blood pressure
- Variable body temperature alternating from fever to chills
- Increased clamminess and paleness of the skin
- Cyanosis (bluish color) around lips, nail beds, and in extremities
- Labored and irregular respirations
- Death rattle (noisy respirations)
- Restlessness and anxiousness

Physical changes one to two weeks before passing:

- The body temperature may decrease by one degree.
- Blood pressure lowers.
- Pulse becomes irregular. It may be 80 then 129 in a matter of minutes.
- Increased sweating.
- Skin color changes; you may notice a bluish tint in fingers and toes and around the lips.
- Changes in breathing. Death rattle sound due to the increased congestion.
- You may notice a lot more sleeping and disorientation.

A couple of days to hours before passing:

- Increased energy.
- Cheyne Stoke breathing, rapid breaths followed by periods of no breathing.
- Mottled skin with bluish purple patches.

This period of time can be called the "transition" because the patient may ask for things she has not asked for in days such as a favorite food or to see a specific relative or friend. She may become alert and speak in short conversations when she has not spoken a full sentence for several days. There is often a spiritual energy that is noted without a physical explanation in this change. This energy may allow the chance to have a requested conversation, to answer a phone call from a family member with whom he or she has not yet talked, and to give some advice to a sibling or child as a way of passing advice or a "blessing" to the next generation. Although common, not all patients experience this transitional time.

Helpful tips:

When the patient appears to be hallucinating, calm reassurance is soothing to the patient. Educate the family the ways in which to respond to a dying patient by holding his or her hand and talking in a soft voice. People recovering from a comatose state recall being able to hear.

As death approaches:

Generally a patient becomes unresponsive at some time prior to death. His or her eyes might be half open, but not able to focus on objects. Peace or fears of facing death may be evident during this transition. Opportunities to say, "I am sorry, I forgive you, thank you, I love you and good-bye" may provide an easier transition through this dying period.

While no two patients are alike, there are some common signs of impending death. It is likely the following signs indicate that death is imminent:

• Confusion
• Death Rattle
• Bluish coloring of extremities
• Shallow respirations with mouth breathing
• Weak and thready pulse

Suggestions to work through grief and loss

- Acknowledge that grief is real.
- Be gentle on yourself.
- Stay busy. Get involved in a volunteering group, take a walk in nature, meditate, and find a grief support group in your area.
- Do the things you have wanted to do.
- Write about your feeling in a journal.
- Surround yourself by loved ones.
- Carve out time to spend with friends. Meet at a coffee shop, practice yoga, companionship.
- Laughter is the best medicine.

Remember, you are not alone!

The most beautiful people we have known
are those who have known defeat, known suffering,
known struggle, known loss and found their way
out of the depths. These persons have an appreciation,
sensitivity, an understanding of life that fills them
with compassion, gentleness, and a deep loving concern.
Beautiful people do not just happen.

-Elisabeth Kubler-Ross

Grief and loss

According to Kubler-Ross, from her book, *On Death and Dying*, there are five stages of grief, the series of emotional stages that someone experiences when faced with impending death or other extreme losses. The five stages are: denial, anger, bargaining, depression and acceptance. These stages are not experienced by everyone and do not come in a particular order.

What to do when they are gone?

Grief and loss sets in but everyone experiences it differently. You may feel sad, depressed or cry a lot. You may wonder if these feelings are normal. Don't be harsh on yourself. Grief work takes time and patience, depending on your culture, faith or past experience with loss;this process is unique to the individual.

Grief may manifest itself physically. You may lose your appetite or sleep a lot.

It helps to see grief as a journey.

Some helpful hints:

- Stay busy but allow time to reflect. Look through photo albums, meditate, and talk about your loved one.
- Express your feelings. Cry and laugh, don't hold back.
- Be creative. Paint, draw, make music, listen to music, and pick up a wood carving class or glass staining.

- Go for long nature walks. It is amazing what nature does to your psyche.
- Join a grief support group in your area.
- Create a memory book with pictures, memorandum, etc…
- Honor special events like birthdays, anniversaries, and holidays by creating something special. Sharing stories, lighting a candle, buying a present for them or whatever feels good to you.
- Nurture your body and soul. Eat healthy, exercise and meditate.

Take time to remember your loved one. Share stories with friends and this in turn will give them permission to share stories with you. People try to avoid talking about the deceased one and feel awkward starting a conversation in order not to upset you. Talking to others lessens the feeling of being alone.

Getting over the pain of grieving takes time but if you answer yes to the questions below you may want to find professional help.

- Am I using drugs or alcohol to cope?
- Do I feel like ending my life?
- Am I not eating well?
- Do I feel responsible for the death?
- Is my mood affecting my work or other relationships?
- Do I feel sad most of the time?
- Do I have nightmares often?
- Am I having trouble expressing my feelings?

Individual, family or group counseling may be beneficial to you.

The grieving process may be more complicated and involved when you experienced a traumatic death, the death of a child, have experienced multiple losses including divorce, have a limited support system, issues left unresolved with the deceased.

Helping children cope with loss

Children grieve differently.
Don't treat children as small adults.

Children between birth and two:

May notice that a parent is missing. They may not be aware of the death but they can sense emotional changes. They may be more irritable, have feeding, sleeping and elimination changes.

Children between three and five:

They have a limited concept of death. They don't believe that the person is gone forever. They repeatedly ask the same questions. They are able to show sadness for short periods of time. They may regress like sucking their thumb, wetting the bed; they need a greater sense of security. Don't disturb their routine.

Children between six and 10:

Are aware the deceased one is not coming back. They seem to be moving in and out of intense feelings; they don't have long periods of grief. They may have angry outbursts and decline in school. They are not prepared for the length of the grief process. They are in need of trustful and honest information.

Pre-adolescents and adolescents:

They emotionally separate themselves from their families. They don't talk about their feelings and may be involved with destructive behavior like drugs and alcohol. They may have angry outbursts and have feelings of depression. Children seem to be in the pressure cooker at this age, having to perform academically and socially. It is particularly important to seek counseling in this age group.

How to talk to children about loss and grief:

- Be honest and truthful. This fosters security.
- Encourage them to talk openly and ask what they already know.
- Create a safe place where the child can show their emotions openly.
- Ask questions to clarify how they are feeling.
- Keep their developmental stage in mind.
- Keep the routine.
- Allow them to show their feelings.

You can:

- Watch their play to find clues.
- Reading books about death or acting out a puppet show helps them process the event.
- Ask them what they know and what they want to know.
- Spend quality time with them.

- Tell them why you are sad, be honest.
- Grief support groups provide valuable information for children, teens and families.
- School counseling may be beneficial.

According to the Kubler-Ross model, children may exhibit the same stages.

For example:

- **Denial**

Children feel the need to believe that the deceased parent will come back. Example: "Mom or Dad will come back."

- **Anger**

Children feel the need to blame someone for their sadness and loss. Example: "I hate Mom for leaving us."

- **Bargaining**

In this stage, children feel as if they have some say in the situation if they bring a bargain to the table. This helps them keep focused on the positive that the situation might change, and less focused on the negative, the sadness they'll experience after the death. Example: "If I do all of my chores maybe Mom or Dad will come back."

- **Depression**

This involves the child experiencing sadness when they know there is nothing else to be done, and they realize they cannot bring the deceased back. The parents need to let the child experience this process of grieving because if they do not, it only shows their inability to cope with the situation. Example: "I'm sorry that I cannot fix this situation for you."

- **Acceptance**

This does not necessarily mean that the child will be completely happy again. The acceptance is just moving past the depression and starting to accept the death. The sooner the parents start to move on from the situation, the sooner the children can begin to accept the reality of it.

The Dash

I read of a man who stood to speak
At the funeral of a friend.
He referred to the dates on his tombstone
From the beginning...to the end.
He noted that first came the date of his birth,
And spoke of the following date with tears,
But said what mattered most of all,
Was the dash between those years.
For that dash represents all the time
That he spent alive on Earth
And now only those who loved him
Know what that little line is worth.
For it matters not, how much we own,
The cars, the house, the cash,
What matters is how we live and love
And how we spend our dash.
So think about this long and hard,
Are there things you'd like to change?
For you never know how much time is left
That can still be rearranged.
If we could just slow down enough
To consider what's true and real,
And always try to understand
The way other people feel.
And be less quick to anger
And show appreciation more,
And love the people in our lives
Like we've never loved before.

If we treat each other with respect
And more often wear a smile
Remembering that this special dash
Might only last a little while.
So when your eulogy is being read
With your life's actions to rehash,
Would you be proud of the things they say?
About how you spent your dash.

— Author Unknown

I retrieved this piece from Ben Matthews's funeral
– a tragic young death of bacterial pneumonia.
(Born November 4, 1979- died February 6, 2013.)

References

Callahan, M. & Kelley, P. (1992). *Final Gifts: Understanding the Special Awareness, Needs and Communications of the Dying.* NY: Bantam books.

Care Guide, Hospice of the Valley, 2013

Hopkins, Jeffrey Ph.D, *His Holiness the Dalai Lama Advice on Dying*, 2002, Atria books

Karnes, B (1986). *Gone from My Sight*. Depoe Bay, OR: Author.

Kübler-Ross, Elisabeth. *On Death and Dying*. New York: Scribners, 1997.

rctclearn.net/documents/2012 *RCTCLEARN Professional Catalog*.pdf, retrieved 08/2013.

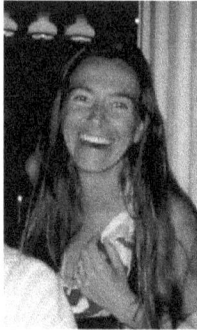

About the Author

Gerlinde Debie-Millette, RN, has risen through the ranks of healthcare from EMT to Unit Coordinator to RN. It took a decade to receive her Nursing Degree raising a family by herself working part-time, attending school full-time and being a mother in between the gaps.

This book was born after working as a Hospice Nurse for 18 months and being faced with the questions from family and patients about death and dying. Her experience and knowledge led her to produce this book with the aim of informing families about the realities they face caring for a dying person, while offering ideas to help everyone involved to make the experience more satisfying for patients and family involved.